LOW CARB MUG MEALS COOKBOOK

Top 50 Ketogenic Style, Low Carb Mug Meals For One That Busy People Will Love!

By
Katya Johansson

COPYRIGHT © 2016 BY KATYA JOHANSSON.
ALL RIGHTS RESERVED.

TABLE OF CONTENTS

1. Chocolate Hazelnut Mug Cake 1
2. Carrot In A Mug 2
3. Almond With Coconut In Mug 3
4. Lemoncoconut Muffin 4
5. Healthy Strawberry Mug Cakes 5
6. Deliciouscaramel Mug Cake 7
7. Pumpkin Pie Chocolate Chip Mug Cake 8
8. Tasty Flax Muffin 9
9. 2 Minute Tasty Cake 10
10. Flaxseed With Vanilla In Mug 11
11. Tasty Nutella Mug Cake 12
12. Huevos Rancheros Egg Whites Mug 13
13. Apple Banana Oatmeal In A Mug 14
14. Tasty Mug Cheesecake 15
15. 5 Minute Amazing Paleo Chocolate Cake 16
16. Tasty Pumpkin Coffee Cake In A Mug 17
17. Lemon Tasty Muffin In A Mug 19
18. Healthy Apple Crisp In A Mug 21
19. Pumpkin Muffin In A Mug 22
20. Amazing Mug Recipe 23
21. Banana French Toast In A Mug 24
22. Tasty Salsa Meatloaf In A Mug 25
23. Spinach And Cheddar In A Mug 26
24. Peanut Butter Mug Cake 27
25. Wonderful Mug Recipe 28
26. Mac And Cheese In A Mug 29
27. Butter Chicken Pot Pie With Naan Crust 30
28. Oreo Tasty Cake With Nutella 33
29. Chocolate Nutella Mug Cake &Strawberries 35
30. Tasty Caramel Mocha Mug Cake 37
31. 5 - Min Gooey Chocolate Mug Cake. 38
32. Delicious Mug Recipe 40
33. Red Velvet Mug Cakes 42
34. Tastu Coconut, White Chocolate & Pecan Mug Cakes 44
35. Cinnamon Roll Mug Muffin 45
36. Lemon Mug Cake 46
37. Flaxseed With Cocoa Powder 47
38. Coconut Flour With Honey 48
Regular Chocolate Mug Cake 49

39. Coconut Mug Cake... 50
40. Tasty Paleo Chocolate Protein Mug Cake......................... 51
41. Healthy Amazing Almond Meal 52
42. Tasty Microwave Cake 53
43. Healthy Dessert 54
44. Healthy Carrot Cake In A Mug 55
45. Low Carb Mug Cookie.. 57
46. Healthy Pumpkin Chai Mug Cake 59
47. Healthy Mug Cookie 61
48. Healthy Cinnamon Mug Recipe 63
49. Tasty Egg Omelet In A Mug.. 64
50. Healthy Pumpkin Oatmeal 65

1. Chocolate Hazelnut Mug Cake

Ingredients

- 2/3 glass hazelnuts, toasted (and cleaned, in the event that you need)
- 3 tbsp cocoa powder
- 2 tbsp granulated erythritol (I utilized Swerve)
- 1 tsp baking powder
- pinch of salt
- 1/4 glass overwhelming cream
- 2 tbsp hazelnut oil (or softened spread or coconut oil)
- 1 big egg (Or Aquafaba – egg replacement)
- 1/4 tsp hazelnut or vanilla extract

Method

1. Grind hazelnuts in food processor.
2. Put into a medium dish.
3. Speed in cocoa powder, erythritol, preparing powder and salt.
4. Blend in cream, oil, egg and hazelnut.
5. Distribute between 2 mugs and microwave each for around 1 minute. Expel

2. Carrot In A Mug

Ingredients

- 2 tablespoons ground flaxseed
- 1 egg
- 1 tablespoon coconut flour
- 3 tablespoons heavy cream
- pinch salt
- 1/4 teaspoon baking powder
- 1 teaspoon cinnamon fluid stevia
- 1/2 teaspoon pumpkin pie flavor (optional)
- 1/4 cup ground carrot
- optional: vanilla cream cheddar icing

Method

1. Whisk all Ingredients together in a coffee cup.
2. Microwave 2 minutes and 30 seconds.
3. Top with icing if wanted.
4. Enjoy!

3. Almond With Coconut In Mug

Ingredients

- 3 tablespoons almond flour
- 1 tablespoon coconut flour
- 1/4 teaspoon preparing powder
- 1/8 teaspoon salt
- 1 huge egg
- 1 teaspoon avocado oil

Method

1. Combine almond flour, coconut flour, baking powder, and salt in a microwavable coffee cup.
2. Include egg and avocado oil. Mix well with a fork.
3. Microwave on high for 1 minute.
4. Expel the biscuit from the cup utilizing a spread blade and cut in half.

4. LEMONCOCONUT MUFFIN

INGREDIENTS

- 1 egg
- 1 tbs. spread (dairy free, utilize coconut oil)
- 3 tbs. unsweetened coconut chips
- 1/2 piling tbs. coconut flour (utilize less for more moist cake)
- 1/2 doonk THM Brand Stevia (or 8 drops of NOW fluid stevia)
- 1/8 tsp Lemon Flavor from Frontier
- 1/8 tsp pure vanilla extract
- a little pinch of salt
- 1/8 tsp preparing pop
- 1/8-1/4 tsp apple juice vinegar

METHOD

1. In an extensive mug, blend the greater part of the Ingredients exceptionally well with a fork.
2. Place in the microwave for 1/2 minutes.
3. Evacuate or eat in the mug.

5. Healthy Strawberry Mug Cakes

Ingredients

For the cakes:

- 2 Tbsp margarine
- 2 Tbsp granulated sugar substitute
- ¼ glass almond flour
- 1 Tbsp coconut flour
- 1 egg
- ¼ glass pureed strawberries
- ½ tsp baking powder
- ½ tsp vanilla extract
- salt

For the Strawberry Whipped Cream

- ½ glass natural overwhelming whipping cream
- 2 Tbsp pureed strawberries
- 1 Tbsp granulated sugar substitute

Method

To make the cakes:
1. Melt the margarine in a microwave safe dish (or in a little pot on the stove). Include whatever is left of the cake Ingredients and mix to combine.

2. For cupcakes: Divide hitter between 4 little silicone cups or paper preparing cups. Microwave every one of them four on a plate for 1 minute.
3. Test with a toothpick, if still not done, microwave for an extra 30 seconds.
4. For mugs: Divide hitter between two coffee cups. Microwave for 90 seconds. Test for doneness, include a few minutes as fundamental. Don't overcook!
5. To prepare in the stove: Bake at 375 degrees (F) for 18 - 20 minutes, on the other hand until a toothpick embedded in the middle tells the truth.

FOR THE STRAWBERRY CREAM:
1. In a medium dish, whip the heavy whipping cream until becomes hard. Join the strawberry puree and sweetener. Fold the strawberry blend delicately into the whipped cream. Spoon or pipe onto the mug cakes.

6. Delicious Caramel Mug Cake

Ingredients

- 1 Tbsp ghee or margarine, liquefied
- 3 Tbsp coconut sugar
- 1 Tbsp almond margarine, daintily liquefied
- 1 vast fed egg
- 1/4 tsp vanilla
- 1/2 tsp lemon juice
- 1/4 cup almond flour
- 1/4 tsp preparing pop
- 1/4-1/2 tsp Celtic Sea Salt (to taste)

Method

1. In a little bowl, combine the ghee (or spread) and sweetener.
2. Include the almond spread, egg, vanilla, and lemon juice until well combined.
3. Include the almond flour, preparing pop, and salt and blend to thoroughly fuse.
4. Separate the player uniformly into two mugs or ramekins and microwave for 1 minute 20 seconds.
5. Serve finished with spread or ghee.
6. Optionally you can prepare these biscuits (in a ramekin) at 350 F for 15-17 minutes or until cooked through.
7. Oil the mug or ramekin with ghee or spread, if craved, to be ready to expel the biscuit from the mug or present with a spoon.

7. Pumpkin Pie Chocolate Chip Mug Cake

Ingredients

- 1 egg, beaten
- 1 tablespoon ground flaxseed
- 1 tablespoon coconut flour
- 2 tablespoons pure pumpkin (not pie filling)
- 1 tablespoon unsweetened almond milk
- salt
- 1/4 teaspoon preparing powder
- 1/2 teaspoon pumpkin pie flavor
- 1/2 teaspoon vanilla fluid stevia
- 1 tablespoon without sugar chocolate chips (I utilize Lily's image)
- optional: genuine whipped cream or dairy free whipped cream

Method

1. Whisk all Ingredients together, with the exception of chocolate chips, until smooth.
2. Mix in the chocolate chips.
3. Empty blend into a 6 ounce ramekin or coffee cup.
4. Microwave 1 minute and 30 seconds or until a toothpick in focus is clean.
5. You can likewise utilize the oven and heat this at 375 degrees for 10-15 minutes.

8. Tasty Flax Muffin

Ingredients

- 1 teaspoon margarine
- ¼ glass flax feast
- ½ teaspoon baking powder
- 2 tsp Splenda
- 1 teaspoon cinnamon
- 1 egg

Method

1. Melt margarine in microwave-accommodating coffee cup
2. Include dry Ingredients
3. Include egg
4. Blend completely
5. Microwave 1 minute or until biscuit is set.

KATYA JOHANSSON

9. 2 Minute Tasty Cake

Ingredients

- 1/4 glass Truvia Baking Blend
- 1/2 glass almond flour
- 3 tbsp unsweetened cocoa powder
- 1/8 tsp baking powder
- 1/2 tsp heating pop
- 1/4 tsp salt
- 2 tbsp coconut oil
- 1 egg
- 2 tbsp heavy whipping cream

Method

1. Combine all Ingredients in a dish until the blend is even furthermore, smooth (no bumps).
2. Pour 1/4 of the blend into a mug and microwave for 2 minutes.
3. Refrigerate remaining player for some other time!

10. Flaxseed with Vanilla in Mug

Ingredients

- 1/4 glass ground flaxseed
- 1 tsp cinnamon
- 1/2 tsp baking powder
- 1 pinch salt
- 1 entire egg
- 1 tsp immaculate vanilla extract
- 3-5 drops fluid stevia or a pinch of powdered stevia

Method

1. Put the greater part of the Ingredients into a standard-sized coffee cup (or larger...but not littler).
2. Blend! Blend! Blend!
3. Put coffee cup in the microwave.
4. Microwave for 1 minute.
5. Turn it over. Give it a couple taps...it will in the long run slide out!
6. Cut it up...enjoy it with margarine, nut spread, dunked in tahini!

11. Tasty NUTELLA MUG CAKE

INGREDIENTS

- 4 tbsp flour
- 1/4 tsp baking powder
- 1/4 glass Nutella
- 3 tbsp fat free drain

METHOD

1. Join all Ingredients into a larger than average mug. Blend with a little race until player is smooth. Cook in microwave for around 1 minute.
2. Sharp blade embedded ought to tell the truth and top of cake ought to look done instead of gooey. On the off chance that cake is not cooked in one minute, add an extra 20 seconds. Give cake a chance to cool in mug totally before eating.

12. HUEVOS RANCHEROS EGG WHITES MUG

INGREDIENTS

- 1/2 glass
- egg whites
- 2 Tbsp.
- Reduced-Fat Shredded Mexican 4-Cheese Blend or
- Monterey Jack Cheese
- 1 Tbsp. prepared to-serve genuine bacon pieces
- 1/8 tsp. bean stew powder if wanted
- 1 Tbsp. zesty dark bean and corn tomato salsa or green taco sauce

METHOD

1. Spray within a huge microwave-safe mug with nonstick cooking Spray. Mix together eggs, 1 tablespoon cheddar, bacon, and stew powder in mug with a fork.
2. Microwave mug on HIGH 1 minute. Mix; microwave 30 seconds longer on the other hand until eggs are set. Sprinkle with residual 1 tablespoon cheddar; top with salsa.

13. Apple Banana Oatmeal in a Mug

Ingredients

- 1/2 glass snappy cooking oats
- 1 tbsp ground flax seed
- 1 egg
- 1/2 glass milk
- 1/3 of a banana, pounded
- 1/4 tsp cinnamon
- 1/2 of an apple, slashed
- 2 tsp nectar

Method

1. Include oats, flax, egg and drain in a mug. Blend well with a fork. Include banana, cinnamon, apple and nectar. Blend again until completely joined.
2. Cook in microwave on high for 2-3 minutes. Cushion with a fork.
3. Mix in a little drain or yogurt or nut-spread if wanted.

14. Tasty Mug Cheesecake

Ingredients

- 2 tablespoons sugar
- 2 tablespoons fat free sharp cream
- 3 tablespoons low fat cream cheddar
- teaspoon lemon juice
- ¼ teaspoon vanilla extract
- ½ egg, beaten soft (egg substitute works as well)

Method

1. Blend in (if wanted) 1 vanilla wafer
2. In a little bowl combine sugar, acrid cream, cream cheddar, lemon pinch and egg until all around joined
3. Microwave on high for 1 minute
4. Open microwave entryway for 20 seconds, close, and microwave again for 45 seconds
5. Remove from the microwave, let cool for 10 minutes, then exchange to the ice chest for around 2 hours
6. Present with a vanilla wafer on top

KATYA JOHANSSON

15.5 Minute Amazing Paleo Chocolate Cake

Ingredients

- 1/2 tablespoons coconut flour
- 2 tbsp. cocoa powder
- 1/2 tablespoons almond flour (or supper)
- 2 tablespoons oil (walnut, canola, olive, or coconut)
- 2 tablespoons crude nectar
- 1 egg
- 1/2 teaspoon vanilla extract
- salt
- cinnamon

Method

1. Combine the greater part of the Ingredients in a little mug. Mix and blend. Place in the microwave for 60 seconds.
2. The highest point of the cake will be moist and gooey (my most loved part!) and the base of the cake will be more cake like. Top with chocolate chips in the event that you wish. Enjoy!

16. Tasty Pumpkin Coffee Cake in a Mug

Ingredients

Cake:
- 1 Tbsp spread
- 2 tbsp sugar
- 2 tbsp pumpkin puree
- vanilla extract, few drops
- 1/4 C All Purpose flour
- 1/8 tsp baking powder
- pinch of salt
- pinch of ground cloves

Streusel:
- 1 tbsp margarine
- 2 tbsp flour
- 1 tbsp cocoa sugar
- 1/4 tsp cinnamon

Method

1. In a mug soften 1 tbsp of margarine in microwave, around 5 seconds. You try not to need it liquefied, simply delicate. Blend in 2 tbsp of sugar and blend until very much joined. Mix in pumpkin, vanilla (only a small piece, we're talking drops), flour, baking powder, and pinch of salt and cloves; blending until simply joined.

Utilize the back of your spoon to smooth it out in the base of the mug.
2. In a different, little bowl, combine 1 tbsp of spread, 2 tbsp of flour, 1 tbsp of chestnut sugar, and 1/4 tsp cinnamon. Utilize your fingers to pinch the spread and blend it in with alternate Ingredients. When it begins to look like uneven sand (appealing, eh?) and all Ingredients are joined, pour on top of cake hitter in mug.
3. Cook in the microwave for 50-80 seconds relying upon your microwave. At 1 minute, my microwave cooks it flawlessly. It will look marginally set on top. You would prefer not to overcook it and things have a tendency to get revolting quickly in the microwave. I propose cooking it 50 seconds, and after that in 10 second interims checking after each interim until done.

17. LEMON Tasty MUFFIN IN A MUG

INGREDIENTS

- 1 egg
- 2 tablespoons flax seed supper
- 1 tablespoon coconut flour
- On the other hand 3½ tablespoons Trim Healthy Mama baking mix
- ½ lemon, pinchd (or 2 tablespoons lemon juice)
- 1 tablespoon margarine
- ½ teaspoon poppy seeds
- salt
- 3 dashes Stevia Extract, or your sweetener to taste
- ½ teaspoon baking powder
- 2-3 drops lemon key oil (I adore NOW mark)
- 2 cup brilliant flax dinner
- 1 cup coconut flour (or another 2 measures of flax dinner or 2 mugs almond dinner)
- 2 tablespoons poppyseeds or chia seeds
- ¾ teaspoon salt
- 2 tablespoons preparing powder
- ½ teaspoon THM Stevia Extract

METHOD

SINGLE MUFFIN INSTRUCTIONS:
1. Mix all Ingredients in a mug or a little bowl.

KATYA JOHANSSON

2. Blend truly well to ensure that your margarine and egg are uniformly joined.
3. Heat in the microwave for 50 seconds or something like that, or in the oven at *350 in 3 general biscuit glasses.

EXPERT MIX INSTRUCTIONS

1. Mix every single dry fixing in a jug.
2. To set up a biscuit in a mug, include ¼ measure of dry blend (1/3 glass on the off chance that you utilized all flax or almond teast/flax), one egg, juice of ½ a lemon, 1 T of margarine, and two or three drops of lemon crucial oil.
3. Blend well, to combine the spread and egg.

18. HEALTHY APPLE CRISP IN A MUG

Ingredients

- 1 little apple, peeled and cut into slight cuts
- 2 tbsp brisk oats
- 2 tbsp flour
- 1 tbsp cocoa sugar (or 1 bundle of stevia)
- 1 tbsp margarine
- ¼ tsp cinnamon
- salt

Method

1. Peel the apple and cut it. I find that more slender cuts cook uniformly in the microwave. Place cuts in a microwaveable mug or little bowl. Microwave for 60 seconds.
2. In the meantime, joined the rest of the Ingredients and disintegrate together with a fork.
3. Mix the cooked apples and after that sprinkle the fixing on top.
4. Microwave for 30 seconds. Mix and after that microwave for an extra 30 seconds.
5. Permit to cool for 5-10 minutes and afterward beat with frozen.

19. PUMPKIN MUFFIN IN A MUG

INGREDIENTS

- 1 egg
- ½ tsp. vanilla extract
- 1 tsp. coconut oil
- 1 tbsp of pureed pumpkin
- 2 tbsp ground flax
- 2 tbsp coconut flour
- ½ tsp. of cinnamon
- a dash of ground cloves
- a pinch of salt
- Stevia to taste
- 1-2 tbsp. of cream cheddar

METHOD

1. Blend wet Ingredients (aside from cream cheddar)
2. Put half of player into lubed dish
3. Layer in the cream cheddar
4. Top with whatever remains of the hitter
5. Heat at 350 for 12-17 minutes

LOW CARB MUG MEALS COOKBOOK

20. Amazing Mug Recipe

Ingredients

- 1 egg
- 1/2 tablespoons milk
- Salt
- Ground dark pepper
- 1/4 of a bagel (or comparative measure of French bread, and so on.)
- 2 teaspoons cream cheddar
- 1/2 cut prosciutto or ham
- New thyme leaves or crisp cleaved chives
- Dijon mustard

Method

1. Beat egg and milk together with a fork in a coffee cup, including salt and pepper to taste. Divide bread into dime-size pieces; mix in. Include cream cheddar; mix in. Tear or cut prosciutto into little pieces; add to blend. Sprinkle with thyme.
2. Microwave on high until done, around 1 minute 10 seconds. Trim with mustard and crisp thyme or chives.

21. Banana French Toast in a Mug

Ingredients

- 2 cuts entire wheat bread, cut in solid shapes
- 1 egg
- 4 tablespoons almond milk
- 2 tablespoons fruit purée
- 2 teaspoons cinnamon
- 1 teaspoon vanilla
- 1/2 banana, cut
- maple syrup

Method

1. Layer a large portion of the bread solid shapes into a coffee cup. Top with 1/2 of the banana cuts. Layer with the rest of the bread solid shapes and top it off with whatever is left of the banana.
2. In a little bowl whisk the egg, almond milk, fruit purée, cinnamon what's more, vanilla together. Pour over the highest point of bananas and bread. Place mug in microwave for 2 minutes on HIGH.
3. Expel from microwave and top with syrup.

22. TASTY SALSA MEATLOAF IN A MUG

METHOD

- 4 oz = 115 g natural ground meat from grass-sustained dairy animals
- 1/4 cup = 60 ml = 1 oz = 30 g shredded cheddar
- 3 tablespoons hand crafted or other sans sugar, food added substance free salsa
- 1/4 teaspoon natural onion powder
- 1/4 teaspoon (or to taste) grungy ocean salt

METHOD

1. Combine all Ingredients in a little bowl. Blend with a spotless hands until it is very much blended.
2. Place the blend into 8-ounce (230 ml) or bigger microwave-safe mug.
3. Microwave at 250 watts for 6–8 minutes. Check after a few minutes and conform the aggregate cooking time as per your microwave oven. Try not to cook too long, generally the meat turns out to be as well dry.
4. Let cool to a normal temperature and serve.

23. Spinach and Cheddar in a Mug

Ingredients

- ½ cupsliced solidified spinach, defrosted and depleted
- 1 egg
- 1cup milk
- 1 cup shredded cheddar
- 1 cup cooked bacon, sliced (optional)
- salt and pepper, to taste

Method

1. In the case of utilizing crisp spinach, place it in mug with 2 tablespoons of water. Spread with a paper towel and microwave on high for one minute. Expel from microwave and empty the water and fluid out of spinach completely.
2. In the case of utilizing solidified spinach, ensure it is totally defrosted and depleted and add it to the mug.
3. Split the egg into the mug with the spinach and include the milk, cheddar, bacon (if utilizing), and salt and pepper. Blend until completely joined.
4. Spread and microwave on high for 3 minutes, or until completely cooked.

24. Peanut Butter Mug Cake

Ingredients

- 2 tablespoons coconut flour
- ¼ teaspoon baking powder
- 1 egg
- 2 tablespoons regular shelled nut butter
- 1-½ tablespoons liquefied coconut oil
- 1-½ tablespoons maple syrup (or other fluid sweetener)
- 1 tablespoon coconut milk (or almond milk)
- ¼ teaspoon vanilla extract
- optional: chocolate chips

Method

1. In a little bowl whisk together coconut flour, and baking powder.
2. Include egg, nutty spread, coconut oil, maple syrup, coconut milk and vanilla and blend completely to combine.
3. Fill into a vast mug and microwave on high for around 2 ½ minutes.
4. Begin checking at around 2 minutes. Let it sit for a couple minute before eating.

25. Wonderful Mug Recipe

Ingredients

- a big mug
- a fluid measuring glass
- a 1/3 glass dry measuring cup
- elbow noodles
- some pre-shredded cheddar
- Water.
- shredded cheddar for minute macaroni and cheddar

Method

1. Put 1/3 measure of elbow noodles into your mug. Include 1/2 measure of water to it. Make certain to utilize a fluid measuring cup to quantify your water. What's more, by inadequate, I mean barely short of 1/2 glass. Essentially you will microwave this blend until the water has vanished. In my microwave this takes around 4 minutes. Microwave it for 2 minutes to begin, then blend. At that point one more minute, and mix once more. At that point a last minute, and the water ought to be absorbed. If not, microwave more.
2. Blend in your milk and cheddar, and microwave for a last 30-60 seconds. Mix exceptionally well to mix everything together into a smooth sauce, and enjoy. We attempted grinding our own particular cheeses and the sauce turned out more slender. In that case I included 1/8 teaspoon of cornstarch to the milk.

26. Mac and Cheese in a Mug

Ingredients

- 1/3 cup little macaroni elbow noodles
- an inadequate 1/2 cup water
- a meager 1/4 glass milk
- 1/2 cup pre-bundled finely shredded cheddar

Method

1. Put the macaroni and the water into a mug. Microwave on full power for 2 minutes. Mix. (Note: the water will bubble over a tad, that is fine)
2. Microwave for one more minute. Mix.
3. Microwave for a fourth minute, and afterward verify that all the water has been consumed. If not, microwave more, until it is gone.
4. Mix in the milk and shredded cheddar and microwave for a last 30- 60 seconds. Mix well, and enjoy.

KATYA JOHANSSON

27. BUTTER CHICKEN POT PIE WITH NAAN CRUST

INGREDIENTS

FOR THE NAAN TOP:
- 1 teaspoon dynamic dry yeast
- 2 teaspoons granulated sugar
- 2 cups in addition to 2 tablespoons generally useful flour, in addition to additional to clean
- 1 teaspoon salt, in addition to additional to top
- 1 teaspoon baking powder
- ¼ glass Greek yogurt
- 2 tablespoons olive oil
- 2 tablespoons margarine, liquefied, to best
- Cilantro, to beat

FOR THE BUTTER CHICKEN:
- 1½ glasses Greek yogurt
- Juice of 1 lemon
- 2 tablespoons garam masala
- 2 tablespoons cumin
- 1 tablespoon ground turmeric
- 1 teaspoon paprika
- 1 teaspoon Kosher salt
- ½ teaspoon cinnamon
- 2 lbs. boneless skinless chicken thighs, cubed
- 4 tablespoons (1/2 stick) margarine
- 2 tablespoons oil

LOW CARB MUG MEALS COOKBOOK

- 1 big white onion, diced
- 4 cloves garlic, minced
- 2 tablespoons ginger, minced
- 1 (14.5 oz) can diced tomatoes
- 1 jalapeno pepper, seeded and minced
- ½ glass chicken stock
- 1½ glasses solidified blended vegetables, defrosted
- 1 glass cream
- 1 tablespoon tomato glue

METHOD

1. Begin by setting up the Naan mixture. In a glass measuring cup, join the dry yeast, 1 teaspoon sugar, and ¾ glass warm water. Let it sit for 10 minutes, or until frothy. Then, filter the flour, salt, residual 1 teaspoon of sugar and baking powder into a huge dish.

2. At the point when the yeast is prepared, blend the Greek yogurt and olive oil into the yeast blend. Fill the dry Ingredients and blend. Whenever the mixture is about framed, utilize your hands to blend and ply until a delicate batter shapes. Cover and let ascend in a warm zone for 2 hours.

3. While you hold up, set up together the chicken marinade. Join the Greek yogurt, lemon juice, garam masala, cumin, turmeric, paprika, salt, and cinnamon in an extensive compartment. Include the chicken thigh pieces and blend well to coat. Cover and refrigerate for no less than an hour.

4. Following 60 minutes, melt 4 tablespoons spread with 2 tablespoons oil in an extensive skillet over medium warmth. Include the diced onion and saute until mellowed, blending frequently. Include the garlic and ginger and cook until fragrant.

5. Include the diced tomato, jalapeno, chicken, and chicken marinade, and cook for 10 minutes. Include the chicken stock and heat to the point of boiling, and afterward lessen to a stew. Stew, revealed, for 30 minutes.
6. Blend in the vegetables, cream, and tomato glue and keep on cooking for 5 minutes.
7. Preheat the stove to 400 degrees F. Shower 6 stove safe mugs or one meal dish with cooking shower.
8. Fill the mugs or meal dish with the Butter Chicken. Put aside.
9. On a daintily tidied surface, turn out the batter. Distribute into 6 break even with pieces and delicately extend to cover the highest points of the mugs.
10. Tenderly press to the sides of the mugs to follow.
11. Prepare until brilliant, around 15 minutes.
12. Brush with dissolved margarine and sprinkle with salt and cilantro, if wanted. Serve warm.

28. Oreo tasty Cake with Nutella

Ingredients

- 1/4 Cup All Purpose Flour
- 1/4 Teaspoon Baking Powder
- salt
- 2 Tablespoon Granulated white sugar
- 2 Tablespoon vegetable oil
- 1/4 Cup Milk
- one piled Teaspoon of Nutella
- 4 Oreo rolls pounded generally

Method

1. In a little bowl, blend generally useful flour, preparing powder and salt
2. In a different dish, include sugar, vegetable oil, drain and whisk until sugar breaks down
3. Include Nutella and speed until Nutella breaks up totally in the milk blend
4. Empty the wet Ingredients into the dry Ingredients and combine
5. This hitter is dainty when contrasted with the normal cake player
6. Presently crease in 2 pulverized Oreo rolls in the hitter
7. Wash a microwave safe coffee cup and don't wipe/dry it. This is done to keep it sodden from inside.
8. Pour the cake hitter in a microwave safe coffee cup until it is 3/4 full.

9. Include remaining 2 pulverized Oreo rolls on top of the hitter. So top in just off to 3/4 to abstain from spilling
10. Microwave on high (power setting 800 W) for 95 seconds. In the event that your microwave power setting is diverse you have to alter + or - 10 seconds. Check the cake following 60 seconds, 75 seconds and 90 seconds.
11. Unique formula says microwave at powder setting 750 W for 65 to 70 seconds. My cake was done at 95 seconds at 800 W power setting
12. Cool totally and present with chocolate Ganache or whipped chocolate icing

29. CHOCOLATE NUTELLA MUG CAKE &STRAWBERRIES

INGREDIENTS

- ¼ C. + 1 T. Oat Flour
- ¼ t. Baking powder
- Pinch of Salt
- 2 T. Cocoa Powder
- 4 T. Coconut Palm Sugar
- 1 Egg
- 3 T. Coconut oil, liquefied
- 3 T. Almond or Coconut Milk
- 2 T. Nutella
- 1½ T. Hot Coffee or Water

FOR THE WHIPPED CREAM:
- ¼ C. Strong Coconut Cream(usually shapes on the highest point of a jar of
- coconut milk)
- 1 T. Nectar
- 3 vast Strawberries, Chopped
- Additional Nutella, for sprinkling on top

METHOD

1. Include the oat flour, baking powder, salt, cocoa powder, and coconut palm sugar to a vast mug and combine with a fork.

2. Include the egg and coconut oil to the mug and blend in with the fork.
3. Include the milk and blend in well.
4. Place the Nutella in the focal point of the player and pour the hot coffee or water over the top.
5. Microwave for around 1 minute and 25 seconds (more or less depending on how solid your microwave is).

FOR THE CREAM:

1. Whip the coconut cream and nectar together with an electric blender for 2-3 minutes. Fold in the slashed strawberries.
2. Place on top of marginally cooled mug cake.
3. Sprinkle with more Nutella, if required.

30. Tasty Caramel Mocha Mug Cake

Ingredients

- 3 tbsp + 1 tsp all-purpose flour
- 1/4 tsp baking powder
- 1/2 tbsp unsweetened cocoa powder
- 1 tsp coffee powder
- 3 tbsp fat free drain
- 1/2 tbsp + 1/2 tbsp salted caramel sauce
- 1/2 tbsp vegetable oil
- extra salted caramel sauce for sprinkling
- whipped cream for topping, optional

Method

1. Include flour, baking powder, cocoa powder, coffee, milk, 1/2 tbsp caramel sauce and vegetable oil into a larger than usual microwave-safe mug. Blend with a little race until player is smooth and no irregularities remain.
2. Include remaining 1/2 tbsp of caramel sauce and whirl it into the player, cautious not to totally blend it in.
3. Cook in microwave for 1 minute. Top of cake ought to be dry. Let cake cool before including whipped cream and sprinkling more caramel sauce.

31. 5 - min Gooey Chocolate Mug Cake.

Ingredients

- 1/4 glass all-purpose flour
- 2 tablespoons unsweetened cocoa powder
- 2-4 tablespoons coconut sugar
- salt
- 1 little egg
- 3 tablespoons coconut milk (or your most loved milk)
- coconut whipped cream, for serving
- 3 tablespoons coconut oil, liquefied
- 1 teaspoon vanilla extract
- 1/2 - 1 ounce semi-sweet chocolate
- 1 tablespoon brewed coffee

Method

1. Lightly grease a microwave safe mug with cooking spray. To the mug add the flour, cocoa powder, coconut sugar and a pinch of salt. Whisk it all together with a fork. Add the egg, coconut milk, coconut oil and vanilla. Use a fork to whisk the batter together until just combined.
2. Try to make sure you have incorporated all the flour off the bottom of the mug. Lightly break up the chocolate and place it in the center of the mug. Drizzle the coffee overtop the batter. Place in the microwave and microwave on full power for 1 minute and 30 seconds to 2 minutes. I have a 1200 watt microwave and found 1

minute and 30 seconds was perfect. Allow the cake to cool 1 minute and then dollop with coconut whipped cream and chocolate shavings. Enjoy right away, warm! Oh, and grab a cold glass of milk too!

32. Delicious Mug Recipe

Ingredients

- 1 tbsp plus 2 tsp cocoa powder
- 3 tbsp spelt flour (or any gluten free plain flour)
- 1/8 tsp salt
- 2 tsp evaporated cane juice or sugar if you aren't avoiding completely
- 1/4 tsp baking powder
- pinch stevia OR 1 more tbsp sugar
- 2-3 tsp coconut oil or vegetable oil
- 3 tablespoons coconut milk (or milk of your choice)
- 1/2 tsp pure vanilla extract
- 1/4 cup of peanut or cashew butter
- 4-8 tsp pure maple syrup
- 2 tbsp cocoa powder
- 4 tsp milk of choice
- 3/4 tsp pure vanilla extract

Method

1. Mix the dry ingredients together
2. Add the liquid ingredients and mix well
3. Transfer the mixture to a mug or ramekin
4. Microwave on high for 30-40 seconds until cooked through OR cook in 180/gas 4 oven for about 14 minutes.
5. Whilst it is cooking mix up the frosting ingredients by popping in a food processor, or you can mix by hand, and place on top of the cooked cake.

LOW CARB MUG MEALS COOKBOOK

6. Enjoy straight from the mug!

33. Red Velvet Mug Cakes

Ingredients

Mug Cake:
- 1 1/2 steamed beets from vacuum pack
- 2 tbsp water
- 1 cup almond flour
- 1/3 cup Swerve Sweetener
- 2 tbsp coconut flour
- 1 tbsp cocoa powder
- 2 tsp baking powder
- Pinch salt
- 2 eggs
- 1 tbsp lemon juice
- 1/2 tsp vanilla extract

Cream Cheese Frosting:
- 2 ounces cream cheese, softened
- 2 tbsp whipping cream, room temperature
- 3 tbsp powdered Swerve Sweetener or other powdered erythritol
- 1/4 tsp vanilla extract

Method

1. For the cakes, puree beets and water together in a food processor or blender until smooth.

LOW CARB MUG MEALS COOKBOOK

2. In a medium bowl, whisk together almond flour, sweetener, coconut flour, cocoa powder, baking powder and salt.
3. Stir in beet puree, eggs, lemon juice and vanilla extract.
4. Divide between 4 mugs and cook on high in the microwave for 1 to 1 1/2 minutes, depending on how gooey you want it.
5. For the frosting, combine cream cheese, whipping cream, sweetener and vanilla and beat until smooth. Pipe or spread onto warm mug cakes.

34. TASTU COCONUT, WHITE CHOCOLATE & PECAN MUG CAKES

Ingredients

- 2 Tbsp butter, melted
- 3 Tbsp granulated sugar substitute
- 1 Tbsp coconut flour
- ¼ cup almond flour
- pinch of salt
- ½ tsp baking powder
- 1 egg
- 3 Tbsp unsweetened almond milk
- 1 tsp vanilla extract
- 2 Tbsp shredded unsweetened coconut
- 1 Tbsp chopped pecans
- 2 Tbsp white chocolate chips

Method

1. In a medium-sized microwave safe bowl, melt the butter if you haven't already. Then add the rest of the ingredients and stir to combine thoroughly. Spoon the batter into 2 mugs, or 4 small paper baking cups.
2. Microwave for 1 minute on high if using the baking cups, 1 minute and 30 seconds if cooking both mugs. Check for doneness and if still liquid in the center microwave for 10 second increments until just set. Serve warm.

35. Cinnamon Roll Mug Muffin

Ingredients

- 1 egg
- 1 tablespoon coconut flour
- 1 tablespoon ground flaxseed
- 1/4 teaspoon baking powder
- 1 teaspoon ground cinnamon
- 1/4 teaspoon ground cloves
- 1/4 teaspoon ground nutmeg
- 1/4 teaspoon vanilla extract
- 2 droppers full liquid cinnamon or vanilla stevia
- 1/4 cup water
- Icing
- 1 tablespoon coconut butter
- 1 tablespoon water
- 1/4 teaspoon pure stevia extract

Method

1. Whisk egg in a bowl then stir in the rest of the ingredients until completely combined.
2. Spray a coffee cup with nonstick cooking spray or grease and pour batter into mug.
3. Microwave for 1 min and 30 seconds, or up to 2 minutes in needed.
4. Remove from mug in desired or enjoy as is.

36. Lemon Mug Cake

Ingredients

- 1 egg
- 2 tablespoons lemon juice
- 2 tablespoons heavy cream
- 1/2 teaspoon lemon liquid stevia
- 2 tablespoons coconut flour
- 1/4 teaspoon baking powder
- pinch salt

Method

1. Whisk the egg, lemon juice, cream and stevia together in a small bowl.
2. Stir in the coconut flour, baking powder and salt.
3. Microwave 1 minute to 30 seconds or until toothpick in center comes out clean.
4. Top with whipped cream if desired!

37. Flaxseed with Cocoa Powder

Ingredients

- 1 tablespoon flaxseed, ground
- 1 egg
- 2 tablespoons unsweetened cocoa powder
- 2 tablespoons unsweetened almond milk
- dash salt
- 1/4 teaspoon baking powder
- sweetener of choice (I use liquid stevia 1/2 teaspoon)
- 1 ounce sugar free chocolate bar (I use Lily's Sweets brand)

Method

1. In a small bowl, whisk chocolate cake ingredients together,
2. Pour into a 6 ounce ramekin or mug.
3. Insert the 1 ounce piece of chocolate to the center of the mug.
4. Microwave for 1 minute or up to 20-30 seconds more depending on your microwave.
5. Enjoy immediately!

38. COCONUT FLOUR WITH HONEY

INGREDIENTS:

- 3 Tablespoons of coconut flour or almond flour.
- 3 Tablespoons of cocoa powder
- 2 Tablespoons of honey (optional, I typically don't use honey. You can add a teaspoon or two of Stevia if you like super sweet stuff.)
- 2 Tablespoons of oil (I use coconut oil, but any other kind or melted butter will do)
- 1 Egg
- 1 Teaspoon of vanilla extract
- 1 Tablespoon of coconut or almond milk
- 2 Tablespoons of 70% cacao or higher dark chocolate pieces

METHOD

1. Put all of the dry ingredients in a mug or bowl. Mix.
2. Add the wet ingredients. Mix.
3. Microwave for two minutes.

4.

Regular Chocolate Mug Cake

Ingredients

- 4 Tablespoons of flour
- 4 Tablespoons of sugar
- 4 Tablespoons of cocoa powder
- 1 Egg
- 1 Teaspoon of vanilla extract
- 3 Tablespoons of milk
- 3 tablespoons of oil

Method

1. Put all of the dry ingredients in a mug or bowl. Mix.
2. Add the wet ingredients. Mix.
3. Microwave for three minutes.

39. Coconut Mug Cake

Ingredients

- 1 heaping Tbsp coconut flour
- 1 heaping Tbsp cocoa powder
- 1 Tbsp almond milk (or coconut)
- 1/2 Tbsp honey
- 1 tsp pure vanilla extract
- 1 egg

Method

1. Combine all ingredients together in a microwave safe mug and mix well. Microwave for 1 minute and 30 seconds to 2 minutes until cooked.

40. Tasty PALEO CHOCOLATE PROTEIN MUG CAKE

Ingredients

- 3 tbsp almond meal (ground almonds)
- 1 tbsp cocoa
- 4 tbsp chocolate brownie whey protein
- 2 tbsp coconut sugar or sugar alternative
- 1/4 tsp baking powder
- 1 whole egg
- 1 egg white
- 2 tbsp melted coconut oil or butter
- 2 tbsp water

Method

1. Add all of the dry ingredients to a bowl and mix well before adding the wet ingredients and stirring until combined.
2. Divide between 1-2 microwavable dishes or mugs and microwave for 1-2 minutes until cooked – I recommend cooking it for 1 minute and then for 20 seconds at a time, checking in between (mine took 1 minute 20 seconds).
3. Either devour your chocolate cake from the mug or run a spatula around the mug and tip it out onto a plate – cover with yoghurt mixed with cocoa and a little sweetener or peanut butter sauce (as described above), or anything for that matter!

41. Healthy Amazing Almond Meal

Ingredients

- 1/2 cup almond meal
- 1/4 tsp baking soda
- 1/4 tsp pumpkin pie spice

Then add the wet ingredients:
- 2 TBSP local honey (if you use raw honey, heat it a bit first; Pure maple syrup or agave will work, too)
- 2 drops real vanilla
- 1 egg
- 3 TBSP pumpkin (from a can - this is what makes it so moist)

Method

1. 1 heaping TBSP dried goji berries (optional; dried cranberries would be nice, too)
2. I stirred again, making sure I'd stirred all the almond flour up off the bottom of the mug.
3. I put it in the microwave for 1 minute and 50 seconds.

42. TASTY MICROWAVE CAKE

INGREDIENTS

- 1 package cake mix
- 1 package any other flavor cake mix

METHOD

1. Mix 1 package Angel Food cake mix with any other flavor cake mix (I like chocolate!). Store in an airtight cup in your pantry.
2. When the craving hits, just mix 3 tbsp. cake mix with 2 tbsp. water in a coffee mug, and microwave on high for 1 minute.

KATYA JOHANSSON

43. Healthy Dessert

Ingredients

- 8 oz cup of Cool Whip Free
- 1 oz box of S/F Fat Free Vanilla Instant Pudding
- .3 oz box of S/F Orange Jello

Method

1. Make Jello as specified in Method on box.
2. Stir in the dry pudding mix.
3. Mix well.
4. Add 8 oz cup of Cool Whip Free.
5. Mix well (mixer or whisk)
6. Transfer to 6 cups (1 cup each)
7. Freeze or refrigerate for at least 3 hours.
8. Enjoy!

44. Healthy Carrot Cake in a Mug

Ingredients

Cake:
- 1 egg
- 2 tablespoons mashed banana
- 1 baby carrot, shredded
- 2 tablespoons almond flour
- 2 teaspoons stevia
- 1 tablespoon Greek yogurt
- 1 teaspoon pumpkin pie spice
- a pinch of baking powder

Cream Cheese Frosting:
- 1/8 cup tofu
- 1/4 cup Tofutti cream cheese
- 1/4 teaspoon vanilla extract
- 1 teaspoon stevia

Method

2. Mix all cake ingredients in a mug
3. Microwave for 1-2 minutes
4. Remove cake from mug and chill in freezer while you make the frosting

5. Blend all of the frosting ingredients together until smooth
6. Slice cake in half, add frosting inside, on top and garnish with extra carrot shreds, walnuts and cinnamon

45. Low Carb Mug Cookie

Ingredients

- 1 tbsp butter
- 3 tbsp almond flour
- 1 tbsp erythritol
- 1 pinch cinnamon
- 1 egg yolk
- 1/8 tsp vanilla extract
- 1 pinch salt
- 2 tbsp sugar free chocolate chips

Method

1. If you're using an oven to cookie this mug cookie, preheat it to 350°F.
2. Melt a tablespoon of butter in a small pan and let it brown a little. This will enhance the flavor of your mug cookie!
3. Brown butter
4. Combine this browned butter with 3 tablespoons of almond flour. If you're almond flour is a little coarse, feel free to pulse it in a food processor to make it a little more fine.
5. Add in erythritol and cinnamon.
6. Then add your egg yolk, vanilla extract and salt.
7. Add yolk
8. Add your sugar free chocolate chips (did you know you can make your own?!). Stir to combine.
9. Add chocolate chips

10. Spray a mug, cup or ramekin with some cooking oil and place your cookie dough in. Flatten it out to ensure even cooking.
11. Press into ramekin
12. Microwave on high for about a minute or bake in the oven for about 10 minutes.
13. Let it cool for a few mins and then dig in!

46. HEALTHY PUMPKIN CHAI MUG CAKE

INGREDIENTS

FOR THE MUG CAKE:
- 2 Tbsp butter
- 1 egg
- 2 Tbsp chai tea, brewed strong
- 2 Tbsp granulated sugar substitute
- ¼ cup almond flour
- 2 Tbsp coconut flour
- ¼ cup pumpkin puree
- ½ tsp baking powder
- 1 tsp ground nutmeg
- 1 tsp ground cinnamon
- pinch of salt

FOR THE WHIPPED CREAM:
- ¼ cup heavy whipping cream
- 1 Tbsp granulated sugar substitute
- pinch of cinnamon

METHOD

FOR THE MUG CAKES:
1. Melt the butter in a microwave safe bowl. Add the egg, tea, sugar substitute, almond flour, coconut flour,

pumpkin puree, baking powder, nutmeg, cinnamon, and pinch of salt. Stir well and divide between two mugs or 4 paper baking cups. Microwave for one minute. Test and microwave for another 30 seconds if necessary. If still not firm, try another 30 seconds, but be careful not to overcook. Cool slightly before topping with whipped cream.

For the whipped cream:

2. Combine the cream, sweetener, and cinnamon in a small bowl and whip until firm. Serve over the still warm mug cakes and eat immediately. If not eating immediately, let the cakes cool completely before adding the whipped cream and then store in the refrigerator.

47. Healthy Mug Cookie

Ingredients

- 1 tbsp butter
- 3 tbsp almond flour
- 1 tbsp erythritol
- 1 pinch cinnamon
- 1 egg yolk
- 1/8 tsp vanilla extract
- 1 pinch salt
- 2 tbsp sugar free chocolate chips

Method

3. If you're using an oven to cookie this mug cookie, preheat it to 350°F.
4. Melt a tablespoon of butter in a small pan and let it brown a little. This will enhance the flavor of your mug cookie!
5. Brown butter
6. Combine this browned butter with 3 tablespoons of almond flour. If you're almond flour is a little coarse, feel free to pulse it in a food processor to make it a little more fine.
7. Add in erythritol and cinnamon.
8. Eryth and cinnamon
9. Then add your egg yolk, vanilla extract and salt.
10. Add yolk
11. Add your sugar free chocolate chips (did you know you can make your own?!). Stir to combine.

12. Add chocolate chips
13. Spray a mug, cup or ramekin with some cooking oil and place your cookie dough in. Flatten it out to ensure even cooking.
14. Press into ramekin
15. Microwave on high for about a minute or bake in the oven for about 10 minutes.
16. Let it cool for a few mins and then dig in! Enjoy alone or with a scoop of low carb ice cream

48. HEALTHY CINNAMON MUG RECIPE

INGREDIENTS

- 2 oz cream cheddar, softened
- 1 egg
- stevia drops, splenda, or other no calorie sweetener to taste
- cinnamon
- 1/2 scoop of protein powder (I utilized Quest Vanilla, however you could utilize any brand and any flavor – simply watch carb tallies!)

METHOD

1. Combine and put in the microwave until done in the center (1 minute + 20 seconds in my microwave)
2. Melt margarine on top and enjoy!

KATYA JOHANSSON

49. TASTY EGG OMELET IN A MUG

INGREDIENTS

- cooking Spray
- 2 eggs
- 1 tablespoon diced broiled red peppers
- ¼ cup spinach
- 1 tablespoon feta cheddar
- 1 teaspoon cut green onions
- pepper to taste

METHOD

1. Spray within coffee cup with cooking shower.
2. Add eggs to cup, utilizing a fork, blend until the burdens are combined.
3. Include broiled red pepper, spinach, feta cheddar, green onions, and pepper to taste.
4. Tenderly mix together.
5. Add coffee cup to the microwave and cook on high for 1 minute and 30 seconds.
6. Expel the mug and let sit for 1 minute.

50. Healthy Pumpkin Oatmeal

Ingredients

- 2 eggs, beat
- 1/3 glass moved oats
- 1 tbsp chia seeds
- 1/4 tsp cinnamon
- Pinch salt
- 1/4 glass skim milk
- 1/4 glass canned pumpkin
- 1 glass of natural skim milk

Method

1. Join ingredients through salt in a mug and blend well.
2. Microwave mug at half power for around 4 minutes, checking focus to see that all egg is cooked through.
3. Present with 8-ounce glass of natural skim milk and a optional sprinkle of maple syrup.

Made in the USA
Las Vegas, NV
04 April 2022